# 10 Minutes Methods To Achieve Weight Loss After 50 Or Menopause

## Lose 20 Pounds, Feel Great & Look More Attractive

A STEP-BY-STEP 10 MINUTES EXERCISE AND RECIPE GUIDE OF 5 INGREDIENTS FOR PEOPLE AFTER 50 OR MENOPAUSE WHO WANT TO LOSE WEIGHT, IMPROVE HEALTH AND LOOK ATTRACTIVE IN 2 WEEKS

PATRICK BRADLEY

limited to your doctor, attorney, or financial advisor or such other advisor as needed) before using any of the suggested remedies, techniques, or information in this book.

# TABLE OF CONTENTS

# Introduction

Women in the stage of menopause and men and adults above 50 years old typically gain weight due to hormonal changes which makes it difficult to burn calories.

Weight gain increases the risk of diabetes, cardiovascular diseases, osteoporosis, osteoarthritis, cognitive deterioration, dementia, depression, and cancer.

Do you want to lose weight? Look more attractive and, improve health? Would you like to be a weight loss ambassador and inspire your family and friends?

If your answer is yes then this eBook is definitely for you. You will discover 10 minutes exercise techniques and delicious recipes you can quickly prepare with minimal ingredients to help you to lose weight in 2 weeks. You will also learn:

- How to set effective goals in your weight loss program

- Clothing to wear to make you look slim & beautiful

- How to lose weight while still enjoying social events

Apply the step-by-step instructions in this eBook to a slimmer, healthier and more attractive body in 2 weeks!

# CHAPTER 1

# Why is it so challenging to lose weight after 50 or after Menopause?

## Little known root causes of overweight

*Causes related to age*

- Basal energy expenditure decreases almost linearly with age this leads to an increased energy balance, especially if food intake is maintained and physical activities reduced[1].

- With age, there is a down-regulation of alpha adrenergic response, which may further cause the development of obesity.

*Causes related to hypoestrogenism*

- Leptin is a protein secreted in adipose tissue that communicates the magnitude of energy reserves to the brain. For the same degree of adiposity, women have higher levels of leptin than men.

---

[1] Milewicz A, Tworowska U, Demissie M: Menopausal obesity -myth or fact? Climateric 2001; 4: 273-83.

- Estrogens intervene in the regulation of this hormone stimulating its secretion. For women of fertile age, the circulating levels of leptin are significantly higher during the luteal phase and its concentration declines after menopause[2].

- Women who live alone tend to gain more weight after menopause.

- In some circumstances, menstrual and reproductive history of women leads to obesity during menopause.

## Why exercise & diet don't always work

Before looking for the other causes for weight gain, you should first analyze the guidelines relate to exercise and diet and try to follow it. Answering the simple questions can help shed some light:

***Are you strictly following a diet and exercise program?*** When planning a weight loss diet, then small details are very important. For example, not following the recommendations of the dietitian-nutritionist may prevent you from achieving your weight loss goals.

***Are you consistent?*** Do you start a new diet every other Monday or go on a new exercise regimen every two months? It is necessary to exercise regularly and consistently, eat healthily and in moderate quantities.

## Why weight gain accelerates after 50 or menopause

There may be additional causes that aren't strictly nutritional.

### *1. Genetics*

Genetic inheritance may predispose you to experience more difficulties in losing weight or keeping the line.

---

[2] Tommaselli GA, Di Carlo C, Pellicano M, Nasti A, Ferrara C, Di Spiezio Sardo A y cols.: Modificazioni dei livelli sierici di leptina in menopausa. Minerva Ginecol 2001; 53: 193-8

However, sometimes, overweight is not "inherited" by genes, but by specific acquired behaviors such as bad eating habits developed since childhood.

## 2. Medications

Certain drugs, such as corticosteroids, antidepressants, and anticonvulsants (antiepileptics), can slow down the rate at which the body burns calories, increase appetite or promote fluid retention.

## 3. Stop smoking

Some people gain weight when they stop smoking. One of the reasons is because nicotine accelerates the combustion of calories. Therefore, the caloric expenditure is lower when one quits smoking.

## 4. Environmental factors

According to the researchers, there are obesogenic environments that stimulate obesity[3].

A study from the University of California (USA) showed that living in an area with many advertisements for fast food increases the risk of overweight and obesity.

## 5. Hypothyroidism

The thyroid gland does not produce enough thyroxine; a hormone that stimulates basal metabolism for suffers from this disorder. This hormone leads to slower metabolism where the body consumes fewer calories and a greater tendency to gain weight or increased difficulty to lose it.

## 6. Chronic stress

Whenever faced with anxiety, the body defends itself by secreting a more significant amount of cortisol, which is a survival hormone that

[3] Papas MA, Alberg AJ, Ewing R, Helzlsouer KJ, Gary TL, Klassen AC: The built environment and obesity. Epidemiol Rev. 2007, 29: 129-143. 10.1093/epirev/mxm009

stimulates the production of glucose and orders the cells to store as much fat as possible, especially in the abdomen área.

### *7. Sleeping badly*

When you sleep sufficient hours, between 7 and 8 hours, the balance is maintained between ghrelin (a hormone that generates an empty stomach sensation) and leptin (a hormone that inhibits the feeling of hunger).

However, lack of sleep causes the concentration of ghrelin to increase and leptin to decrease. Result? After a bad night, you feel hungrier and desire sweets and food with sugar.

## 15 "Healthy Foods" that cause weight gain

You already left aside chocolate, chips and fast food but you still do not lose weight? Those "healthy foods" that you have at your disposal and that you are consuming them are dangerous. According to people, they are healthy, but actually they can make you overweight. Below is a list of those foods.

### *1. Walnuts*

While nutrition, nuts macadamia, are very high in fat. The nut mix is an excellent choice because you can get the nutritional benefits of many varieties in a single snack.

### *2. Granola*

This tasty cereal is composed of oats, sugar, and butter that cause you to gain weight.

### *3. Olive oil*

The fats of olive oil are very healthy and also provide Vitamin E but neither satiate nor add volume to meals. For every extra spoonful of oil a day we add 110 calories, and if it is also used for frying, it loses all its nutritional benefits.

### *4. Peanut butter*

Peanut butter is full of protein and fat, which makes it easier for people to gain weight. One scoop alone contains about 100 calories.

### *5. Avocado*

These delicious green vegetables contain healthy fat. If you always add them to your diet, it's possible to gain weight easily as half an avocado alone contains 140 calories.

### *6. Yogurt*

An enhanced or in the past improved yogurt may contain excessive sugar. Do not hesitate to check the labels if what you are looking for is a healthy option.

### *7. Caesar salad*

Salads are a double-edged sword since ingredients, and excessively caloric condiments are often added, such as the Caesar salad that, in addition to the lettuce, has breaded chicken (chicken + bread + fried) and fried bread dices, all watered with the Caesar salt (made with yogurt). In total 1,000 calories in a single dish. It would be preferable to change the breaded chicken for grilled chicken and croutons of fried bread for toast on the griddle or toaster and change the sauce for aromatic oil or vinaigrette.

### *8. Butter*

Butter contains saturated fat, so it's best to consume it in moderation. A better option is to incorporate ghee (vegetable fat) into your diet. This Indian ingredient is an ultra clarified butter. It is safe to use when cooking at high temperatures, unlike ordinary butter, which will burn. Ghee also has a concentrated flavor so it can be used in smaller quantities when cooking.

### *9. White Bread*

Besides causing weight gain, white bread lacks the fiber and minerals offered by whole grain varieties.

### 10. Whole milk

A simple substitution that makes you gain weight is when you replace skim milk with whole milk. You will also gain weight when you add milk to your coffee.

### 11. Red meats

The steak contains high levels of iron and protein. Fatty cuts contain more fatty meat. These cuts of meat contain more calories though they are also tastier. Avoid rib, chop, New York steak, and sirloin. Red meat is high in cholesterol.

### 12. Cheese

Cheese is one of North America's favorite foods. However, it is high in fat, so consume in moderation.

### 13. Protein bars

Protein bars are intended to be a healthy snack for athletes, but not all are: beware of those high in sugars or carbohydrates and ahead with those that consist of nuts and fruit.

### 14. Sweeteners

Taking them produces a reaction in the intestinal flora that could lead to glucose intolerance.

### 15. Agave syrup

Due to the reluctance around sugar and sweeteners, there are those who resort to other sweetening ingredients such as agave syrup. Its proponents claim that it is less harmful than sugar because, because it contains little glucose, it does not cause insulin spikes. However, what is exceptionally high is fructose, a substance that in large quantities is related to heart problems and obesity (yes, just like sugar ...)

# 30 little known simple tricks to lose weight

We bring you 30 tricks you can implement immediately to lose weight without diet and without requiring much effort.

*Trick #1: Buy blue crockery*

This color helps you to control hunger so that you will avoid excessive food intake. Avoid red dishes, because this tone stimulates appetite.

*Trick #2: Avoid liquids in food*

Drinking water during diet slows down digestion. Once you have finished your meal, wait a few minutes before drinking any kind of liquid.

*Trick #3: Meditate*

This technique helps balance your mind and relax your body. In addition, it reduces stress, which causes hormones to be altered and generate an accumulation of fat.

*Trick #4: Wear comfortable shoes and walk*

When you walk, you burn calories and tone your buttocks, back, and calves. So take advantage of any available time to walk and lose weight.

*Trick #5: Use sugar substitutes*

It does not contain calories, so you will not gain weight.

*Trick #6: Use floral aromas*

According to a study by Dr. Alan Hirsch, director of the Aromas and Flavors Research Foundation in Chicago, 190 men underestimated the weight of women by up to 7% when the women wore a floral perfume.

*Trick #7: Breakfast fruit*

This food stimulates digestion, so your metabolism works in a more efficient way. After the fruit, you can ingest carbohydrates to give you energy.

### *Trick #8: Alcohol with the measure*

Studies show that women who drink alcohol are less likely to gain weight than abstainers[4], because alcohol speeds up metabolism and curbs appetite. Remember to consume in moderation, such as only one glass of red wine a day.

### *Trick #9: Enjoy the aroma of the dishes*

The aroma of the food sends a signal to the brain that you have just eaten food, so a feeling of satisfaction is experienced. Before giving each bite, take a deep breath as it will curb your appetite.

### *Trick #10: Divert your mind*

Wash your teeth after eating. Its good hygiene, and you will also avoid the temptation to eat. If you feel a craving, chew gum or fruit instead.

### *Trick #11: Have a fixed lunch schedule*

Choose an approximate time to eat and try to stick to it. When you eat under the same schedule, you avoid having hunger between meals. Avoid snacks or unhealthy snacks.

### *Trick #12: Improve your food options between meals*

The diversity or variety of food is important. Try to have all kinds of products to obtain a balanced diet. A diet that gives you all the vitamins and nutrients your body needs. Not a single meal every time!

### *Trick #13: Walk whenever you can*

---

[4] Suter PM. Is alcohol consumption a risk factor for weight gain and obesity? Crit Rev Clin Lab Sci. 2005;42:197–227

When you manage to increase your physical activity within your routine, you will be using more energy, and therefore it is easier to lose weight. A pedometer is an excellent resource, it is cheap, easy to use and it also motivates you to keep track of your steps. Not the question is: how can you find opportunities to walk and make walking fun? Next are some examples.

### Example 1: Basic walk for those who start

So that its effects are visible, you must walk one hour a day. This is the time your metabolism needs to start "burning" fats.

- ### How to choose the route?

Take advantage of a known journey from your town or city, but remember that you must go at a constant pace and without stopping to look at shop windows. In total, you must do 4 km in 1 hour. So you will burn at least 230 kcal, although the higher your weight, the more energy you will consume.

- ### Start little by little

First heat 5 minutes, walk briskly 50 minutes more and dedicate the last 5 to cool. Your goal should be to improve little by little and not go farther or faster than someone else.

### Example 2: Intense but controlled walk

If you used to do some physical exercise, you could adapt this type of walk. To do it, you only have to increase the speed in certain sections of the route.

- ### Proposed route

Once familiar with the basic technique of walking, it is time to insert a few minutes of more intense exercise into your route that will help you to spend even more energy. Take shorter steps and more frequently and you will achieve more speed. You can also choose to climb a hill and burn 40% more energy. In total, you must travel 6 km in 1 hour.

- *How to do it?*

Start with 5 minutes of warm-up, walk 35 more at a brisk pace, increase the speed for the next 15 minutes and, finally, spend 5 minutes cooling down.

### Example 3: Combined treadmill to lose weight even faster

It is proven that, if you change your rhythm when exercising, you burn fatter. Once you have acquired a better physical shape, we suggest that in your alternate outings the walk with the soft race.

- *Recommended itinerary*

The objective is to travel 7 km in an hour on a route that allows you to walk and run at the same time. In addition to burning more calories, running will avoid monotony during the journey. You will also define your silhouette since running you put in operation many more muscles.

- *Program well a journey*

Look for possible places where a stop to rest at the right moments.

- *How to do it right?*

After 5 minutes of warm-up, walk very fast or run 10 more minutes, stop to stretch for another 5 minutes, speed up the step 15 more minutes, for another time to do toning exercises, speed up again 15 minutes, and end up cooling.

*Trick #14: Before buying a product, check its label*

It is not about counting each calorie before buying a product. But, what you can do is a quick analysis. Just look at the portion that marks the label for the nutrition fact and the ingredients.

*Trick #15 Look what you put on your plate*

Serve yourself a normal portion and if you're still hungry, repeat. This way it is easier to control the portions of what you are eating. This rule does not apply to fresh vegetables (because you can eat the ones you want).

Eating from the container or the bag makes you lose track of how much you've eaten. Better be on a plate and visualize the quantity.

### *Trick #16: Say no to sugary drinks*

Think about this, when you drink a soda, you are actually taking more than 10 teaspoons of sugar without realizing it. Therefore, avoid soda and always prefer water.

### *Trick #17: Eat more slowly and with attention*

Eating is a pleasure, and it should be enjoyed. Unfortunately, we sometimes forget it and only introduce food to our mouths. Direct your attention to what you eat and taste every bite, improve your satiety, your digestion and prevent weight gain.

### *Trick #18: Paint colors your foods with fruits and vegetables*

Do not forget to eat 5 servings of vegetables daily and 3 to 5 servings of fruit, either fresh or frozen. Include a serving of vegetables at each meal. Fruits are an excellent choice as a dessert and/or as a healthy snack.

### *Trick #19: Have a good breakfast*

Eat a breakfast of 300 calories. A healthy combination of proteins and cereals is what allows you to have a lot of energy throughout the day and what is better, eat less at any time.

### *Trick #20: Eliminate temptations*

Eliminate everything that causes weight gains in your cupboard and replaces them with healthy ones.

### *Trick #21: Healthy meetings*

Instead of hanging out with friends to eat pizza, it's better to cite them in the park for exercise or at least to breathe fresh air.

<u>*Trick #22: Do not eat at dawn*</u>

In the event that you are one of the individuals who get up during the evening, opens the refrigerator and searches for something to "nibble", you should change this propensity for a more advantageous one. You can take a stab at drinking a glass of water.***Some snacks that you can take***

- *1-Homemade popcorn*

Although the popcorn eaten in movie theaters are related to fat, the truth is that you can make healthy and very rich natural popcorn. They are simple to make, very economical and in short, they have nothing to do with packaged popcorn to be made in the microwave.

- *2-Cottage cheese snacks with Cinnamon*

It is a snack rich in proteins and low in calories, with an amount of calcium that can help metabolize fat.

Take half a cup of cottage cheese with cinnamon powder, something that will allow the processing of glucose to be accelerated, preventing the fat from being stored. You can even add apple slices.

- *3-Tuna with wholemeal crackers*

Tuna cannot miss among these healthy snacks. Tuna with wholemeal crackers give you 200 calories and three grams of fiber, considering that it is a great source of omega3 and proteins.

- *4-Kale chips*

The kale, you can consider it a superfood. It is rich in fiber and antioxidants such as quercetin and kaempferol. These compounds help to reduce blood pressure and the risk of colon cancer. 1 cup of raw cabbage provides you with more than 100% of the recommended daily amount of vitamins A, C, and K.

<u>*Trick #23: Make your environment work for you*</u>

Please do not have the freezer full of ice cream. Because although every time you enter the kitchen you are able to resist the delicious flavor of vanilla with macadamia nuts, the day will come when you are sad or tired, and you can not control yourself (your willpower is exhausted), and that day you will eat the whole boat.

### *Trick #24: Do not repeat the same recipes again and again*

Get rid of all the foods you have at home that do not serve to cook any of the 6 meals you have chosen. Go to the supermarket and buy what you lack. When it's time to eat, choose one of the dishes from the recipes in Chapter 3.

### *Trick #25: Find (or hire) someone who requires you to be responsible*

With a personal trainer, you will receive advice and guidance from a professional expert, who will create tailor-made training programs, follow your progress and keep you motivated to achieve your goal. But if you train with a friend, there is a risk that you end up talking rather than training and when you leave the gym, you end up in a bar.

### *Trick #26: Drinking soup*

Add a broth-based soup every day. The soup is especially useful at the start of a meal, as it slows down food and reduces appetite.

### *Trick #27: Green tea*

It can accelerate the burning of calories, possibly through the action of catechins. You can enjoy a refreshing drink without tons of calories.

### *Trick #28: Red sauce*

Tomato-based sauces will in general have less calories and less fat than cream-based sauces. Remember it in your pasta dishes.

### *Trick #29: Eat less meat*

Eating vegetarian meals more often is a good habit to lose weight.

### <u>*Trick #30: Burn 100 calories*</u>

Walk 20 minutes fast, run 10 minutes, clean the house for half an hour ... these small exercises not only burn calories but reduce appetite.

# Chapter 2

# 10 minutes exercise techniques to lose stubborn fats

These techniques are based on performing five exercises in eight series of 15 seconds. After a previous warm-up, the glutes, legs, arms, and abdomen are toned for 10 minutes in total.

They can be done in any place and surfaces and no specialized equipment is needed. In addition, this method allows you to continue losing fat even after you have finished. Here are the five exercises.

## Exercise #1: Squats

*Duration: 2 minutes*

It is the star exercise to work glutes and strengthen them. To optimize its benefits, the professionals aim to separate the legs by the width of the shoulders, pull the ass back and lower without joining the knees and keeping the back straight. Once below the horizontal, get up little by little keeping the position straight. Repeat intensely for 15 seconds and rest the next 10, until the eight series required.

## Benefits

1. They help develop flexibility around the hips when you do them correctly and gradually increase the range of motion.

2. The muscles you use when doing squats are the same ones you used to jump, run and sprint, so you'll have more resistance.

3. Squats burn a lot of calories and stimulate the cardiovascular system.

4. By working the long muscles of the body, the bone density of the spine, hips and legs increases, which helps you to prevent osteoporosis, mainly in women.

5. If you add a certain weight gradually, it is an excellent anaerobic, so your muscle mass will increase.

6. With a good work of repetitions, without needing so much weight, it helps you to tone the glutes, to define them and to give them hardness.

7. They improve the position because when doing a squat, the abdominals and spinal are also exercised, which work as a support to maintain the position of the back.

## Exercise #2: Push-ups

*Duration: 2 minutes*

To gain resistance in the arms, place your hands on the floor at shoulder height, perpendicular. The body is stretched and the tips of the feet rest on the ground, with force. Little by little, lift the body keeping the back and hip in the same line.

## Benefits

1. Increase base strength

2.  Increase bone mass

3.  Increase metabolic rate

## Exercise #3: Burpees

Known as 'the jump of the frog', this exercise raises the heart rate quickly and, therefore, burns fats more easily. What does it consist of? It begins by doing a squat, and the hands are supported in front and on the ground, the body is pushed back into the position of flexion, the body is pushed forward again -recognizing the squat pose- and ends with a jump to stay standing.

## Benefits

1.  Work the whole body

2.  Attacks directly to body fat

3.  Improve your resistance

4.  Strengthening your muscles

5.  Improve cardio

6.  Work the balance

## Exercise #4: Step

*Duration: 2 minutes*

The classic aerobic exercise is retaken in this training. A step or bench is needed and, during the corresponding 15 seconds, one foot is raised and lowered and the other repeatedly.

## Benefits

1.  Improve your cardiovascular performance and the absorption of oxygen by your body.

2. It helps you to reduce your body fat by consuming a large number of calories.

3. Tones buttocks, legs, and hips, one of the areas that most concerns, especially women.

4. Increase the strength and resistance of the muscles in your legs.

5. Improve your flexibility and coordination.

6. It helps you to eliminate daily stress, to relax and to feel more comfortable with yourself.

7. Step choreographies allow you to exercise in a fun and stimulating way.

8. Improve your memory when you have to learn the choreography of the step.

## Exercise #5: Abdominals

*Duration: 2 minutes*

The body is laid down, and the soles of the feet are supported on the ground. With force, the trunk rises until the shoulders touch the knees, without helping the arms and without lifting the feet. Repeat during the established time.

## Benefits

1. Keep the internal organs in a proper position and relaxed state.

2. Produces improvement in intestinal health.

3. You will avoid hernias and protrusions.

4. It will also make you breathe better.

# CHAPTER 3

# 10 Delicious recipes of 5 ingredients you can easily prepare in 10 minutes

## 1-Pumpkin cream

*Total serving size*: 1

*Nutrition per serving*:

- Calories: 38

- Carbohydrates: 2.6g/Dietary: Fiber 0.1g/Fat: 2.9g/Protein: 0.6g

*Preparation and cooking time*: 10 minutes

| Ingredients |
| --- |
| 1 pumpkin |
| 2 onions |
| 2 cloves of garlic |

| |
|---|
| 1 tbsp butter |
| Laminated almonds to decorate |

## Preparation:

1. Cut the pumpkin into pieces and salt and pepper.

2. Bake the pumpkin at 180° C until it is soft.

3. Brown onions over low heat with butter.

4. Fry the previously chopped garlic.

5. Blend the pumpkin with the garlic and onion. Add a little water if necessary, so that the consistency of cream remains.

6. Garnish with the rolled almonds.

## Benefits

- It has a low caloric density, that is, it is ideal for controlling weight because it contains a large amount of water.

- Its beta-carotene protects us from UV rays, so it contributes to the care of your skin.

- It has a high content of vitamin A (100 g of pumpkin contain more than 200% of the recommended intake of this vitamin), which is very beneficial to the eye.

- It also gives you good doses of vitamin C, which helps you fight infections and is a good ally in the colds season.

- Its fiber content helps you to regulate intestinal transit and also favors the pancreas in the control of glucose, which is interesting for people with diabetes.

- It helps you to strengthen the immune system because it is an important source of antioxidants.

- Folic acid-containing help in the protection of heart attacks.

## 2- Baked salmon

*Total serving size*: 1

*Nutrition per serving*:

- Calories: 234

- Carbohydrates: 0g/Dietary Fiber: 0g/Total: Fat 14g/Protein: 25g

*Preparation and cooking time*: 10 minutes

| Ingredients |
| --- |
| 500 g of salmon |
| 1 lemon |
| 1 tsp of dill |
| 1 tsp pepper |
| Capers to taste |

**Preparation:**

1. Grease a baking dish and place the salmon with the skin facing down.

2. Season and add the dill and lemon zest.

3. Bake at 180° C for 10 minutes.

4. Add the capers before serving.

**Benefits**

- Help keep the heart healthy

- It can help to reduce inflammation. It is a powerful food able to end joint pains

- Omega-3 is an important aid in the prevention of cognitive problems

- It can help to reduce the risk of suffering from different diseases in the eyes

## 3- Apple tartlets

*Total serving size*: 2-3

*Nutrition per serving*:

- Calories: 696

- Carbohydrates: 94g/Dietary Fiber: 4.4g/Fat: 30g/Protein: 11g

*Preparation and cooking time*: 10 minutes

| Ingredients |
| --- |
| 3 apples |
| 250 g of puff pastry |
| 2 butter spoons |
| 1 tbsp of brown sugar |

**Preparation:**

1. Cut the peeled apples into thin slices.

2. Stretch the puff pastry, paint with butter and sprinkle brown sugar.

3. Place the apple on the puff made of strips and roll up so that it is a flower shape.

4. Bake at 180° C until the puff pastry is browned.

### Benefits

- Lower cholesterol and blood sugar

- Lower risk of circulatory and heart diseases, lung cancer, and asthma

## 4-Brie cheese toast

*Total serving size*: 1-2

*Nutrition per serving*:

- Calories: 208

- Carbohydrates: 15g/Sugars: 1.7g/Fat: 12g/Protein: 9.3g

*Preparation and cooking time*: 5-10 minutes

| Ingredients |
| --- |
| 1 large onion |
| 1 tbsp butter |
| Bread cut into slices |
| Brie cheese |
| Sliced tomato (optional) |

### Preparation:

1. Split the onion into thin strips

2. Put the butter in a pan and when melted add the onion.

3. Cook over a very slow heat so that the onion does not become dehydrated.

4. Toast the bread, add the brie cheese and on top the cooked onion and some slices of tomato.

**Benefits**

- Brie cheese contains 22.61 grams of protein and does not contain carbohydrates

- It does not contain sugar, contributing 341.90 calories to the diet

- It has vitamins B7, B3, A, and B9. In addition to these properties, brie cheese contains calcium.

## 5- Chia Seed Pudding

*Total serving size*: 1

*Nutrition per serving*:

- Calories: 200

- Carbohydrates: 21g/Fiber: 6.3g/Fat: 8g/Protein: 12g

*Preparation and cooking time*: 10 minutes

| Ingredients |
| --- |
| ½ cup of chia seeds |
| 1 cup of almond milk |
| A pinch of cinnamon |

| |
|---|
| 1 fruit that you like |

## Preparation:

1. For the preparation, you must mix all the ingredients in a bowl and put them in the fridge for 10 minutes. If you wish, you can use the same fruit to decorate your recipe or use nuts.

*<u>Note</u>*: Chia seeds are easy to get in the market will help you with weight loss and will provide you with extra energy.

### Benefits

- It helps you lose weight

- It has valuable fats for the cardiovascular system

- It is an antioxidant for a strong immune system

- It is good for the hair and skin

## 6-Pancakes with protein

*<u>Total serving size</u>*: 2-3

*<u>Nutrition per serving</u>*:

- Calories: 110

- Carbohydrates: 8.2g/Fiber: 1.1g/Fat: 1.5g/Protein: 10.6g

*<u>Preparation and cooking time</u>*: 5 minutes

| Ingredients |
|---|
| ½ cup quick-drying oatmeal |
| 4 egg whites |

| |
|---|
| ½ tsp of sugar |
| ½ of cinnamon |
| Vanilla extract and chopped fruit |

## Preparation:

2.   Add all the ingredients in a bowl, beat with a fork.

3.   Pre-heat a Teflon pan and add the mixture forming a pancake.

4.   Cook until the dough begins to form bubbles on the top, about 1 to 2 minutes with low flame turn it over and cook it for 2 more minutes. Add the chopped fruits and eat. If you wish, you can find more ideas to add protein to your pancakes.

_**Note**_: The pancakes in the morning are the golden dream of breakfast. How to make them healthy and fast is the key to not go over your body weight, you will get 270 calories with 20 grams of protein.

### Benefits

*   Better sources of proteins

*   Provide vitamins and minerals

*   It is based on cereal that gives you slow-digesting sugars, proteins, vitamins, and fiber7- Smoked salmon sandwich

_Total serving size_: 2-3

_Nutrition per serving_:

*   Calories: 470

*   Carbohydrates: 0g/Dietary Fiber: 0g/Total: Fat 28g/Protein: 50g

_Preparation time_: 2-5 minutes

| Ingredients |
| --- |
| 2 slices of smoked salmon |
| 1 tbsp of hummus |
| ½ avocado, chopped |
| ¼ cup sliced tomatoes |
| 2 slices of whole grain bread |

**Preparation:**

1. Add hummus to the top of the bread and add the smoked salmon in layers, then the sliced avocado, onion, and tomato.

*Note*: Sandwiches are the easiest and quickest to prepare in the mornings, either in the week or on weekends at home.

**Benefits**

We have already mentioned the benefits that you can find in the Salmon in recipe #2. The same benefits are applicable to this recipe because it is based on salmon.

# 8-Kitchari

*Total serving size*: 1-2

*Nutrition per serving*:

- Calories: 476

- Carbohydrates: 82g/Fiber: 22g/Fat: 7g/Protein: 22g

*Preparation and cooking time*: 5 minutes

| Ingredients |
| --- |
| |

| |
|---|
| ¼ red lentils |
| ¼ cup of brown rice |
| 1 carrot cut into squares |
| ¼ cup of frozen soybeans |
| 1 cup of water with a pinch of salt |

**Preparation:**

1. Add the lentils, rice, chopped carrots and the cup of water to boiling point. Then, over low heat, wait for it to cook when the water is drying, and add the peas and soybeans. Turn off the heat, let it rest for 5 minutes and season it to your liking.

_**Note**_: This dish, we can say is easy food because it does not take much science in its preparation. Everything is in the fire that you apply to your kitchen.

**Benefits**

- It is a detoxifying and restorative

- decreases the aging of cells

- offers abundant nutrients

- helps eliminate accumulated waste

## 9-Beef Ramen

_Total serving size_: 4

_Nutrition per serving_:

- Calories: 1468

- Carbohydrates: 164g/Fiber: 9.6g/Fat: 22.4g/Protein: 72g

*Preparation and cooking time*: 10 minutes

| Ingredients |
| --- |
| 1 red pepper cut into strips |
| 1 tsp of vegetable oil |
| ½ lb of beef cut into strips |
| 4 Tbsp sweet chili sauce |
| 2 packages of ramen flavored with beef |

## Preparation:

2.  Heat the oil in a pan over low heat.

3.  Add the pepper and cook for 4 minutes or until lightly browned.

4.  Add the meat strips and season with salt.

5.  Cook for 3 minutes.

6.  Reduce the heat and add the sweet chili sauce.

7.  Cook the noodles apart (let them stand in boiling water to cook for 3-4 minutes).

8.  Sprinkle the condiment envelopes on the noodles and stir.

9.  Add the meat and peppers.

10. Serve it hot.

## Benefits

- Good source of iron

- It contains carnitine

- Provides all essential amino acids

- Provides Vitamin B12

- Good for muscles

- Great source of proteins

## 10-Pumpkin noodles with spinach and parmesan

*Total serving size*: 4

*Nutrition per serving*:

- Calories: 404.1

- Carbohydrate: 28.8 g/ Fiber: 6.1 g/Fat: 15.0 g/Protein: 29.6 g

*Preparation and cooking time*: 5-10 minutes

| Ingredients |
| --- |
| 3 medium courgettes |
| 2 Tbsp butter |
| 2 garlic cloves, chopped |
| 2 cups of spinach |
| ¼ cup grated Parmesan cheese |

**Preparation:**

1. Form spirals with zucchini and removes them.

2. Melt the butter in a large skillet over medium-high heat and add the garlic.

3. Cook for 1-2 minutes.

4. Add the zucchini noodles and spinach.

5. Mix gently and cook until the spinach leaves soften.

6. Stir in ¼ cup of Parmesan cheese and mix until the zucchini noodles are coated with the cheese.

7. Season with salt and pepper to taste

8. Remove from heat and serve hot.

**Benefits**

Thanks to the spinach, this dish is an excellent natural resource of vitamins, fibers, and minerals, which, compared to meat, provides few calories and is fat-free.

- The spinach helps you to lose weight

- Promotes transport and oxygen deposition in tissues

- Increase muscle strength

- It favors intestinal transit

- Promotes energy and vitality

- It helps prevent diseases

- It benefits pregnant women and children: due to its content of folic acid (vitamin B9

# CHAPTER 4

# Additional proven weight management strategies

## Strategy #1: Set effective goals in your weight loss program

Having realistic goals in weight loss is essential. How many times have you started a new year or a Monday morning with a resolution like this? "I'm going to exercise every day from now on, no matter what." Or "I'll never eat that chocolate or the desserts again", and "I need to lose five kilos in the following two weeks." Very often, health food nuts have made "unsuccessful" circumstances for themselves, having unreasonable and mistaken assumptions regarding how "perfect" it tends to be, and how much weight they can lose.

The best way to avoid disappointment is to learn to set realistic goals. Many people create goals that are too high, or that are out of reach, rather said at the top of Mount Everest. For example:

- "I have to lose twenty kilos"

- "I'm going to walk fifteen kilometers."

You have to find the objectives that allow you to live with them, and incorporate them into your daily schedule. Here are some examples of unrealistic goals that can sabotage your weight loss efforts, as well as examples of realistic goals that can fuel your weight loss efforts.

### Unrealistic goals

1. Do not eat. From restricting excessively amounts to eating only once a day.

2. Reward yourself the achievements with food.

3. Fix yourself only on the total weight

4. Take your diet as a temporary punishment

5. I will start walking for two hours and so every day.

6. Sleep a little

7. Do not give yourself occasional quirks.

### Realistic goals

1. I will never eat more than 1,000 calories a day. My average daily consumption will be 1,500 calories a day this week.

2. Starting tomorrow, I will walk for 20 minutes four times this week.

3. I'm going to make cookies for sale, and I'm not going to eat or taste any.

4. I will buy cookies for sale, and I will leave them at school on my way home from the grocery store.

5. I'm going to lose five kilos before my meeting with friends next month.

6. I'm going to eat small portions, and I'll take a 15-minute walk four times a week to feel healthier, fitter, and confident for next month's meeting.

Make sure you write your goals. Then read to make sure your lifestyle fits the description of realistic goals. If you cling to the demanding, point to goals that are reasonable or prudent with yourself, then review your thinking and your goals as well.

## Strategy #2: 14 fashion tricks to help you look slim & beautiful

Trick #1: Invest in lingerie

Start from the inside out, because it does not matter how beautiful the clothes you wear if the bra does not project the desired effect. To do this, invest time and money in looking for lingerie that meets the requirements that your chest needs. It's a subtle but powerful change that radically modifies the way you will look.

Trick #2: Respect the proportions

Very few are chosen that have a perfectly harmonious silhouette between upper and lower body, in general, the bodies are very different from each other, some wider up, others with the little-marked waist, others with the hips more voluminous; other very thin, high, low... Hence, the importance of dressing according to your body proportion.

Trick #3: When in doubt, monocolor

It does not matter if you are very thin if you are tall, low; have many curves or large size. The solution of wearing one color (and not necessarily black) is always a good choice, to be able to add the accessories that best fit you.

Trick #4: Dress in three colors

If the monocolor does not go with you, and it is not a question of going dressed in color without looking like a part of Parcheesi, the big key is to dress in three colors and at least two that are neutral.

Trick #5: Use strong tones to your benefit

And we continue with the color keys because they are much more important than you think. It is no longer that you favor one more than another, it is that the way you use them determines the successful outcome or not of your look. You must use dark and strong tones in your favor:

If you have the lower part of the body wider, bet on the most marked tonalities and printed on the top. And vice versa, if you want to boost the lower one, give color to that area and bet on the neutral in contrast.

Trick #6: The power of vertical stripes

Look that there are urban legends about the clothes that feel better, but this is one of the few that is not. It is a proven fact that vertical stripes lighten the silhouette and stylize. This trick applies to all body types.

Trick #7: Choose shoes in nude colors

Although the black is what has more fame, the reality is that those who feel better with almost all looks are a nude color, the closest to the natural tone of your skin. Just as black gives a radical cut on your skin (more in spring than you go without socks), the lighter ones harmonize the silhouette.

Trick #8: Layers and more layers

And by layers, we do not mean clothing on garments, but you play with the textures and lengths of the clothes. If you go in jeans and a T-shirt, add a long jacket, a caftan or kimono also quite long and check the result.

Trick #9: Up (a little) the shot of the clothes

We are not in favor of carrying all the clothes with the high shot, because in jeans, for example, it can do the opposite effect on pronounced hips. However, in cloth pants, your bet is always to raise it a little to mark the waist. And it works for both upper and lower area.

Trick #10: It's not the length of your skirt, it's the fall

Contrary to popular belief, midi and long skirts are perfect for all body types. Thinners should opt for pleats and folds, and those with more curves should opt for stiffer fabrics and straight silhouettes. And very important, that the midi skirt reaches just two spans above the ankle and the long tape covers the feet almost completely.

Trick #11: The ankles in sight

Pay attention! We do not say, Capri or pirate so that pants stylize, the perfect height is, according to experts, two fingers above the bone of the ankle.

Trick #12: An American that stylizes

You can not join the oversize trend if you want to stylize your final look. It is obvious. According to the stylists, it should fit on the shoulders and attention, very important; the sleeve has to fall exactly on the wrist.

Trick #13: The belt is THE KEY

If there is an accessory that you must have as the protagonist of your outfits, that is the belt. Because if you put it on an American, mark waist, without adding to your jeans, power curves, without adding to a very straight dress, magic.

Trick #14: Teach the instep

It seems incredible that it is such a minor detail and so important for the final look. The final trick so that your silhouette lengthens and seems more harmonious, no matter your size, is that the instep opens the shoes.

## Strategy #3: How to lose weight while enjoying social events

### *1- Plan, whenever possible*

If the event is organized at home, you can plan a menu that matches your diet, looking for options that are also attractive to other diners. On the other hand, it is at the home of a trusted friend or relative, you can request to adopt the menu a little or propose a meeting where everyone brings a dish.

### *2- Ask the waiter*

If the food is in a restaurant, as the waiter for healthy options available. You can also the request the chef no to add salt to your menu.

### *3- Value short term vs long term*

Understandably, maintaining good diet habits during social gatherings can be complicated at times, and you may want to give yourself a rare treat occasionally! However, there are ways to go around it. See tip #4 below!

### *4- Control the quantities*

You may not have full control over the menu, but you can certainly restrict the amount of food you consume. Be disciplined not to overeat.

### *5- Stop if you are satisfied*

Eat slowly, chewing properly, tasting and enjoy the food, and know when you should stop.

### *6-Alcohol or food: not both*

After a hard the week at work, it is tempting to indulge in a "cheat meal". The recommendation is to choose between only alcohol and food. Summary of action plans

**Set a deadline**

- Find an inspiration with some festival or date assigned for you. Think about a dress, coat or pants that you presently unfit to wear however might want to wear on a specific date.

Before starting

Use the 10 recipes that are proposed in the chapter 3 to incorporate them into your daily dish, taking into account that these are very effective and balanced. You can also use one of the three types of walks (the 3 examples) according to your physical form. It is advisable to start with the first one and with time you increase the difficulty level.

**Mark your "flying goals"**

Goals in the medium and short term that favor reaching small objectives to give you an extra energy injection like:

- "I'm going to feed myself better, so I'll stop eating cookies mid-morning."

- "I'll run on Tuesdays."

- "I will reduce the beers on Friday afternoon, to one."

**Set markers to see if you're doing things right**

- "I will weigh myself and measure my contours once a week" (Pay attention! Do not obsess, not weigh yourself more times, the fat goes before).

- "I will use some application or pedometer that measures the distance I run".

**Write down the difficulties that you think you will encounter to achieve success**

- "In two weeks I have lunch with my brothers-in-law, and they always make my favorite dish".

- "Next month the child complies, and I have to make several cakes, it is difficult for me not to fall into temptation".

**Propose the solutions to the difficulties that you set before**

- "Within two weeks I have the food with my brothers-in-law": you can bring some original salads for everyone and thus you will have fewer caloric alternatives.

- "Next month the child complies, and I have to make several cakes"

You can substitute cakes for something healthy, rich and fun because it is also important that children learn to eat better and so you will have an alternative. Your creative energy will assist you with saving these circumstances, and you will feel great by the day's end and not have fallen into temptation.

**Example of an action plan**

Establish a goal of weight and moderate physical activity to work on it from here to the next session.

Moderately intense physical activity means you're working to raise your heart rate and sweat a little. You can talk, but not sing.

Examples of moderate exercise are the following:

- Walk at a rapid pace.

- Dance.

- Riding a bike on flat terrain or some hills.

- Take part in sports with your children or grandchildren.

| |
| --- |
| My goals in the next 6 months are:<br>Reach _______ pounds / kilos<br>Perform at least _______ Weekly minutes of moderate physical activity. |

**Actions**

Make a list of 3 actions to perform to lose weight and meet your health goals.

| My goal to lose weight for this program is __________. Date: __________. My goal of time dedicated to moderate intensity physical activity per week is __________ minutes. | |
| --- | --- |
| **Action 1: What am I going to do?** | |
| Where will I do it? | |
| When can I do it? | |
| How long am I going to do it? | |
| What are possible obstacles or challenges? | |
| Solutions to my obstacles or challenges | |
| **Action 2: What am I going to do?** | |
| Where will I do it? | |
| When can I do it? | |
| How long am I going to do it? | |
| What are the possible obstacles or challenges? | |
| Solutions to my obstacles or challenges | |
| **Action 3: What am I going to do?** | |

| | |
|---|---|
| Where will I do it? | |
| When can I do it? | |
| How long am I going to do it? | |
| What are the possible obstacles or challenges? | |
| Solutions to my obstacles or challenges | |

**Completed Actions** Use this chart to help you to see how your actions are doing. Have you completed them successfully? Where can it improve?

| | Action 1 completed? (Yes or No) What worked and what did not? | Action2 completed? (Yes or No) What worked and what did not? | Action3 completed? (Yes or No) What worked and what did not? | Ideas to improve or overcome challenges |
|---|---|---|---|---|
| Today's date:_____ | | | | |
| Today's date: _____ | | | | |
| Today's date:_____ | | | | |
| Today's date:_____ | | | | |

| Today's date:______ | | | | |
| --- | --- | --- | --- | --- |
| Today's date:______ | | | | |